TO LOSE WEIGHT

NO INTERVENTIONS

NO REMEDIES

NO LIES

A Year of Dedication and Reeducation – No Turning Back.

There are moments in life when we recognize the need for deep and lasting change.

It's as if an inner voice whispers that it's time to take the reins, to dedicate ourselves to a journey that will transform us from the inside out.

It's in these moments that we make the decision to commit an entire year to our own re-education, to our search for genuine and lasting well-being.

This book is a guide for that journey, a companion in your quest for a healthier, happier, and more meaningful life.

Entering a year is a unit of time that, when viewed up close, can seem alarmingly long. However, when we look at the bigger picture, a year is just a fraction of the time we have in our lives.

Therefore, the choice to dedicate a year to a journey of re-education and personal transformation is a monumental decision.

It's a statement of commitment, an affirmation that you value your health, your happiness and your potential in a way that deserves extraordinary attention and effort.

This is not just another self-help book, nor a quick-fix manual for short-term problems.

Rather, it's a complete program that spans 365 days, a program that demands your continued dedication and your willingness to embrace lasting change.

This is an invitation to a profound re-education, a transformation that embraces all aspects of your life —

body, mind, and spirit.

We recognize that the journey we propose will not be without challenges.

After all, true transformation is never easy. However, it's the willingness to face these challenges that makes us stronger and leads us to achieve our deepest goals.

We are not looking for temporary solutions, but rather lifestyle changes that will last a lifetime.

We want you to understand that there is no way back - and,

honestly,

you won't want to go back.

Obesity is a multifactorial condition that goes beyond mere aesthetics.

It's intrinsically linked to several serious health problems, including type 2 diabetes, cardiovascular disease, hypertension, sleep apnea, osteoarthritis, some types of cancer and many others.

Furthermore, obesity can have a negative impact on mental health, contributing to depression, anxiety, and low self-esteem.

The quest for quick and drastic weight loss has been a trend, with many fad diets and extreme methods promising immediate results. However, these approaches are typically not sustainable and can be harmful to your health in the long term. In contrast, healthy, natural weight loss focuses on achieving and maintaining a suitable body weight through balanced, long-lasting lifestyle changes.

Here are some reasons for this approach to be so important:

1. Long Term Health:

Choosing healthy, natural weight loss aims to improve your health in the long term. Making sustainable lifestyle choices, like improving your diet and increasing physical activity, not only helps you lose weight but also helps you maintain a healthy weight over time. This reduces the risk of several health problems associated with obesity, such as type 2 diabetes, heart disease and high blood pressure.

2. Safety and Wellbeing:

Extreme diets and rapid weight loss methods can be dangerous to your health. They can lead to nutritional deficiencies, loss of muscle mass, and other harmful side effects. A natural, healthy approach is safer and promotes overall well-being.

3. Sustainability:

Healthy, natural weight loss focuses on making changes gradually and developing sustainable habits. This makes it more likely that people will maintain their new weight over time rather than gaining it back after a temporary diet.

4. Lasting Behavior Change:

This approach emphasizes behavior change over quick fixes. This means people learn to make better food choices and incorporate physical activity into their lives on an ongoing basis, which is critical to long-term success.

5. Self-Esteem and Mental Health:

Healthy weight loss also considers mental health.

Extreme approaches can lead to feelings of failure and low self-esteem when goals are not achieved.

A balanced approach promotes a healthier relationship with your body and food, improving self-esteem and mental health.

6. Example for Others:

By taking a healthy, natural weight loss approach, you can become a positive role model for friends and family. This can inspire those around you to make healthier choices and embrace an active lifestyle.

7. Less Accordion Effect on weight loss:

Fast, extreme diets often result in an accordion effect, in which people lose weight only to quickly regain it. Gradual weight loss is more effective in preventing the accordion effect, as it creates sustainable habits.

8. Education and Autonomy:

By taking a healthy, natural approach to weight loss, people have the opportunity to learn about nutrition, physical activity and how these factors affect their body. This allows them to take control of their own health and make decisions based on information.

In summary, healthy, and natural weight loss is not only an effective approach to achieving a healthy body weight, but it's also crucial for long-term health maintenance.

By making balanced and sustainable choices, you not only improve your physical health, but also promote your mental and emotional well-being.

So, when facing the challenge of weight loss, always remember to prioritize your long-term health and well-being.

Obesity is often assessed using Body Mass Index (BMI), which is calculated using the following formula:

BMI=divide height2(m2) by weight(kg)

Where:

"Weight" is body mass in kilograms (kg).

The "height" is the height in meters (m).

The BMI result can be interpreted as follows according to the categories established by the World Health Organization (WHO):

BMI below 18.5: Underweight

BMI between 18.5 and 24.9: Normal weight

BMI between 25 and 29.9: Overweight

BMI between 30 and 34.9: Grade I obesity

BMI between 35 and 39.9: Grade II obesity

BMI over 40: Grade III obesity

OBESITY CAUSES:

Obesity does not have a single cause, but is the result of the interaction of several factors, including:

Diet: Excessive calorie consumption, especially from foods high in fat and sugar, contributes to weight gain.

Physical Inactivity: Sedentary lifestyles, in which physical activity is limited, are a significant risk factor for obesity.

Genetics: Genetic predisposition can influence the likelihood of developing obesity, but it's not decisive.

Psychosocial Factors: Stress, depression, and other emotional factors can lead to inappropriate eating behaviors.

Environment: The availability of high-calorie foods and limited access to healthy foods can influence eating patterns.

HEALTH IMPLICATIONS:

Obesity is more than an aesthetic concern; it has serious health implications.
Some of the health conditions associated with obesity include:

Type 2 Diabetes: Obesity is a major risk factor for developing type 2 diabetes, a condition characterized by insulin resistance.

Cardiovascular Diseases: Obesity is associated with a greater risk of high blood pressure, coronary heart disease and stroke.

Respiratory Problems: Obesity can lead to respiratory disorders, such as sleep apnea, which affect sleep quality and overall health.

Joint Problems: Excess weight puts additional pressure on joints, contributing to osteoarthritis and other musculoskeletal problems.

Psychological Problems: Obesity can lead to mental health problems, including depression, anxiety, and low self-esteem.

Cancer: Some types of cancer, such as breast, colon, and prostate cancer, are associated with obesity.

Liver Problems: Hepatic steatosis, or non-alcoholic fatty liver disease, is more common in people who are overweight.

CONSULT A HEALTHCARE PROFESSIONAL

Before making any significant dietary or lifestyle changes, consult a doctor or nutritionist. They can help you assess your current health status and create a plan that suits your needs.

THESE ARE THE TESTS YOU NEED TO START YOUR WEIGHT LOSS PROGRAM:

Complete Blood Test: A complete blood count can provide information about overall health, including blood cell counts, kidney and liver function, and blood glucose levels. This can help identify underlying health problems that may affect your ability to lose weight.

Assessment of Thyroid Function: Thyroid problems, such as hypothyroidism or hyperthyroidism, can affect metabolism and make weight loss difficult. A blood test that measures levels of thyroid hormones, such as TSH, T3, and T4, may be indicated.

Lipid Profile: This test evaluates the levels of total cholesterol, HDL ("good" cholesterol), LDL ("bad" cholesterol) and triglycerides. It is important to assess cardiovascular risk and monitor the effects of diet on blood lipids.

Fasting Blood Glucose: Fasting blood glucose measures blood sugar levels after a period of overnight fasting. This can help identify prediabetes or diabetes, which can impact how you approach your diet.

Assessment of Kidney Function: Tests such as serum creatinine and glomerular filtration rate (GFR) are used to assess kidney function. Kidney problems can influence diet and protein intake.

Assessment of Liver Function: Tests such as ALT (alanine aminotransferase) and AST (aspartate aminotransferase) measure liver function. Liver problems can affect the body's ability to metabolize fats.

Blood Pressure Measurement: High blood pressure can be a risk factor for cardiovascular diseases. It's important to measure your blood pressure regularly, as diet can affect your cardiovascular health.

Nutritional Assessment: Consulting a registered dietitian or nutritionist can help assess your current nutritional status, identify deficiencies, and plan a personalized diet.

Basal Metabolism Assessment: In some cases, an assessment of basal metabolism (how many calories your body burns at rest) can be helpful in determining ideal calorie intake for weight loss.

Body Composition Assessment: Measuring body fat percentage, lean body mass, and body mass index (BMI) can help you set realistic weight loss goals.

FRANKNESS AND TRUTH

Thinking before eating any food means considering not only the momentary taste, but also the nutritional value and benefits that each food will bring to your body and your health.

This doesn't mean you should give up all indulgences, but rather that you should find a balance between gastronomic pleasures and healthy choices.

Food awareness involves questions such as:
"Is this food nutritious?"
"How will I feel after eating it?"
"Will this help me achieve my weight loss goals?"
and
"Am I really hungry, or am I just eating out of emotional impulse?"

Remember that it's not just what you eat, but also how and why you eat that plays an important role in your journey. Practicing food awareness can help you avoid impulsive consumption and emotional eating.

"Don't buy what you can't eat."

1. Avoid Temptation: When you fill your home with unhealthy foods or foods that don't align with your weight loss goals, you are creating constant temptation. Having these foods in plain sight makes it harder to resist them, especially in moments of weakness.

2. Promote Healthy Choices: By stocking your pantry and refrigerator with healthy, nutritious foods, you are creating an environment conducive to healthy food choices. You will be more likely to consume these foods when you are hungry or need a quick meal.

3. Save Money: Buying only what you can and should eat helps avoid food waste. Plus, you save money by avoiding spending on unhealthy or unnecessary items.

4. Stay Focused: When you follow the rule of not buying what you can't eat, you are staying focused on your weight loss and health goals. This reinforces your commitment and determination.

5. Simplify Life: An organized pantry and refrigerator aligned with your goals makes life simpler. You don't need to spend time and energy deciding between unhealthy options; your choices are already defined.

6. Build Sustainable Habits: This practice helps to build sustainable eating habits. Instead of relying on willpower to avoid inappropriate foods, you are creating an environment that automatically supports your goals.

7. Strengthen Discipline: Not buying what you can't eat is an exercise in discipline.
Strengthens your ability to make conscious choices and control your eating impulses.

Include Exercise in Your Daily Routine

A Realistic Path to Physical Activity
and Weight Loss

Excitement often leads us to make impulsive decisions, like joining a gym without fully considering our current situation.
This initial excitement can, unfortunately, turn into frustration and discouragement when we realize that we are unable to maintain assiduity in activities.
It's important to recognize that being overweight can make physical activity more challenging at first.
Movements that seem simple to other people can seem difficult and uncomfortable when carrying extra weight.
Therefore, before committing to an intense gym routine, it's wise to take a more gradual and realistic approach to physical activity.
An effective way to start moving is to incorporate exercise into your daily life.

Walking, climbing stairs, cleaning the house and working in the yard are excellent forms of physical activity that can be done at your own pace.

These everyday movements help you build a solid foundation and familiarize yourself with physical activity, preparing you for a more advanced level of exercise at the gym.

It's important to remember that there is no one-size-fits-all approach. Everyone is different, and what works for one person may not work for another.

Therefore, do not compare yourself to others as this can lead to feelings of inadequacy.

As you progress on your weight loss journey and become more comfortable with physical activity, you may want to consider joining a gym.

However, it is crucial not to rush this step. Gradual weight loss, accompanied by a progressive increase in physical activity, can be more sustainable and rewarding in the long term.

Stay Hydrated

The amount of water a person needs per day can vary depending on several factors, including age, gender, physical activity level, climate, and individual health.
However, there is a general recommendation that may be useful as a starting point:

the known
"Recommended Daily Water Intake"
or
"RDI"(Recommended Daily Intake).

The RDI of water for adults
generally
is around 2.7 to 3.7 liters per day,
which is equivalent to
about 8 to 12 glasses of water of 250 ml each.

However, this amount may vary.

Remember that water is essential for many body functions, including temperature regulation, digestion, nutrient absorption, waste elimination, and general organ function.

Dehydration can lead to a range of health problems, including fatigue, dizziness, constipation and even kidney problems.
A practical way to check hydration is to pay attention to the color of your urine.
Light yellow or pale urine is usually a sign of good hydration, while dark or concentrated urine may indicate a need to increase water intake.

Ultimately, it's important to listen to your body and meet your individual hydration needs.

If you are unsure about your specific needs, consulting a healthcare professional can be helpful for personalized guidance.

Drinking water is essential for the body to function properly. Stay hydrated throughout the day, and opt for water as your main drink.

Get Enough Sleep

Adequate sleep is vital for health and weight loss. Try to maintain a consistent sleep routine, avoid stimulants before bed, and create an environment conducive to rest.

Manage Stress and Emotions

Learn stress management techniques such as meditation, yoga, or breathing exercises.
Avoid emotional eating by looking for healthy alternatives to deal with stress.

Monthly Assessment vs. Daily: Balancing the Mindset

Monitoring progress daily can, in fact, generate anxiety and discouragement.
Normal fluctuations in body weight, which can occur due to a variety of factors such as fluid retention, hormones, and digestion, can be disconcerting if observed constantly.
The scale can become a source of stress, leading to an overly critical and negative approach to the weight loss process.
Monthly assessment, on the other hand, allows for a broader, more balanced perspective on progress. It gives the body enough time to respond to changes in diet and physical activity, reducing anxiety associated with daily fluctuations.
The monthly approach encourages patience, acceptance of normal fluctuations and a more realistic and sustainable view of the weight loss journey.

Using the Tape Measure: Beyond Body Weight

In addition to taking a monthly approach, using a tape measure is an excellent way to track progress more comprehensively. While the scale only focuses on total body weight, the tape measure measures changes in the circumference of key areas of the body such as the waist, hips, thighs, and arms. Tape measures are a more accurate representation of changes in body composition, as they can indicate muscle mass gains, body fat reduction, and body shaping, even when body weight may not be changing significantly.
This is especially important for those who are incorporating exercise into their routine, as muscle weighs more than fat.

THE DIET SUMMARY

A Healthy and Balanced Diet Plan

When following a diet plan to achieve your weight loss and health goals, it is essential to adopt a balanced and sustainable approach.

Here's a diet plan that incorporates healthy choices and can help you create a nutritious foundation for your journey:

1. Eliminate Processed Sugar:
Avoid refined sugars such as sucrose and high fructose corn syrup.
Replace white sugar with healthier alternatives, such as raw honey, pure maple syrup or coconut sugar, in moderation.

2. Use Healthy Vegetable Oils:
Opt for unrefined vegetable oils like extra-virgin olive oil, avocado oil, or virgin coconut oil for cooking. Avoid partially hydrogenated oils and processed oils, which are high in unhealthy trans fats.

3. Reduce Red Meat Consumption:
Cut down on red meat and opt for lean sources of
protein such as chicken breast, fish, legumes and
plant-based proteins such as tofu and beans.

4. Eliminate Alcoholic Drinks:
Alcohol is high in calories and can interfere with
making healthy eating decisions.

5. Replace Rice with Quinoa:
Quinoa is an excellent choice as it is rich in protein,
fiber, and nutrients. Replace white rice with quinoa
to increase the nutritional value of your meals.

6. Increase it up with Fruits and Vegetables:
Increase your consumption of colorful fruits and
vegetables at every meal. They are rich in vitamins,
minerals, and antioxidants essential for health.

7. Include Whole Grains:
In addition to quinoa, include other whole grains
such as oats, barley, quinoa, and whole grain bread
in your diet to provide fiber and slow-release energy.

8. Hydrate Yourself Adequately:
Drink water throughout the day to maintain
adequate hydration.
It's important to drink enough water, especially when
reducing your consumption of sugary drinks.

9. Keep controlled portions:
Practice portion control to avoid excess calories.
Use smaller plates and pay attention to your satiety
needs.

10. Plan Meals and Snacks:
Make a weekly meal plan and include healthy
snacks between meals to keep your energy levels
stable.

The phrase

"Don't eat like an ox if you are not one"

succinctly summarizes the importance of understanding and respecting adequate portions in your diet.

People often have a natural tendency to consume larger portions than they actually need, which can lead to excess calories and weight gain.

Here's how you can apply this concept to your weight loss journey:

1. Portion Awareness:
Start by developing an awareness of what constitutes an adequate portion.
This involves learning to recognize the correct serving size for different foods, such as proteins, carbohydrates, fruits, and vegetables.
2. Avoid Oversizing Your Meals:
Avoid the trap of oversizing your meals. Remember that the size of your plate can influence how much you eat. Opt for smaller plates to help control portions.

3. Practice Portion Control:

Practicing portion control is essential. Use measuring utensils, such as cups and spoons, to serve food and ensure you are eating the right amounts.

4. Listen to the Signs of Satiety:

Pay attention to the satiety signals your body sends. Eat slowly, savor each bite, and stop when you start to feel full, not when you are completely full.

5. Avoid Emotionally Eating:

Avoid eating for emotional reasons or in response to stress. Instead, learn to deal with emotions in a healthy way, without turning to food for comfort.

6. Plan Meals and Snacks:

Plan your meals and snacks in advance to avoid excessive hunger, which can lead to larger portions. Keep healthy snacks on hand to avoid impulsive choices.

7. Divide into Smaller Portions:

If you tend to eat large portions, divide your food into smaller portions at the beginning of the meal. This helps control the amount you eat.

8. Appreciate Quality, not Quantity:
Remember that the quality of food is more important than quantity. Prioritize nutritious, balanced foods rather than just focusing on quantity.
9. Take Care of the Desserts Size:
Reduce the size of your desserts or opt for healthier options, such as fresh fruit, natural yogurt, or small portions of dessert occasionally.
10. Stand Firm with the Phrase:
- Whenever you find yourself tempted to overindulge in portions, remember the phrase
"Don't eat like an ox if you are not one."
to maintain control and moderation.

Maintaining an active social life while following a diet may seem like a challenge, but it's completely possible to balance both.

Here are some tips to help you enjoy social gatherings while sticking to your diet:

1. Plan it in Advance:
Before attending social events, plan your meals and snacks in advance. This helps ensure you are nourished and less likely to make impulsive food choices.

2. Communicate with Friends and Family:
Talk openly with friends and family about your diet and health goals. They can be more understanding and offer food options that fit your diet.

3. Choose Restaurants with Healthy Options:
When going out to eat, choose restaurants that offer healthy options on their menus. Many places now have low-calorie alternatives and vegetarian options.

4. Bring a Dish to Contribute:
If you're going to a social gathering where there will be shared food, bring a dish that meets your dietary needs. This ensures you have at least one healthy option available.

5. Make Conscious Choices:
At the social event, make conscious choices regarding food. Opt for smaller portions, avoid fried foods and opt for healthier options such as salads, vegetables and lean proteins.

6. Avoid Overindulging in Alcoholic Drinks:
Excessive alcohol consumption can lead to poor food choices and excess calories. Drink in moderation and alternate with water to stay hydrated.

7. Have a Recovery Plan:
If you end up eating too much at a social occasion, don't be discouraged. Have a recovery plan for the next day and get back to your healthy eating routine.

8. Practice Moderation:
It's important to remember that a healthy diet allows for occasional indulgences. You don't need to avoid all indulgent foods, just consume them in moderation.

9. Focus on the Company, Not the Food:
Focus on company and fun during social events rather than just the food. This can help reduce the temptation to overeat.

10. Maintain Long-Term Balance:
Remember that long-term balance is the key. An occasional less healthy meal or day will not compromise your overall progress.

11. Involve Friends in Active Activities:
Instead of just meeting for meals, plan social
activities that involve exercise, like walks, bike rides,
or dance classes.
12. Track Your Progress:
Keep a record of your progress to stay motivated
and remember your goals.

Remember that a healthy diet is an important part of
your health journey, but it shouldn't stop you from
enjoying your social life.

With planning, communication, and conscious
choices, you can balance both effectively.

RECIPES THAT WILL BE THE BASIS FOR YOUR DIET

REPLACING RICE WITH QUINOA IS A HEALTHY AND NUTRITIONAL CHOICE.

Here's a simple recipe for making quinoa in a similar way to rice:

Ingredients:

1 cup of quinoa
2 cups of water or vegetable broth (for more flavor)
Salt to taste (optional)

Instructions:

Rinse the Quinoa:

Before cooking, wash well the quinoa in cold water. This helps remove quinoa's natural bitter flavor, called saponin.

Drain and Rinse:

Use a fine sieve to drain the quinoa after washing. Make sure the quinoa is completely drained.

Heat a Pan:

In a medium pan, heat a little oil (optional) over medium heat.

Toast the Quinoa:

Add the quinoa to the pan and toast it for a few minutes until it starts to release a nutty aroma. This enhances the quinoa's flavor.

Add Liquid:

Pour 2 cups of water or vegetable broth into the pan. Add a pinch of salt if desired. Increase the heat and bring to a boil.

Cook on Low Heat:

As soon as the water starts to boil, reduce the heat to low. Cover the pan and let the quinoa cook over low heat for about 15 minutes, or until all the liquid is absorbed.

Rest it and Release it with a Fork:

After cooking, remove the pan from the heat and let it rest, covered, for another 5 minutes. This helps to loosen the grains and ensure the quinoa is cooked through.

Serve and Enjoy:

Fluff the quinoa with a fork before serving. Now you have a healthy and versatile base to accompany your favorite dishes, just like you would with rice.

Quinoa is an excellent source of protein, fiber and other essential nutrients, making it a nutritious alternative to rice in your meals.

You can use it as a side dish, in salads, or as a base for main dishes.

Try combining with veggies, lean proteins, and flavorful sauces to create delicious, healthy meals.

You can enhance this recipe by adding potatoes, carrots, peas, whatever you want, for maximum variation.

Season with garlic and onion to enjoy every meal.

EVERY DAY TO REPLACE THE BREAD

LITTLE EGG AND OAT PIE WITH HONEY AND CINNAMON

Ingredients:

1 whole egg
1/4 cup rolled oats (you can adjust the amount to obtain the desired consistency)
Honey to taste
Cinnamon powder to taste
A pinch of salt (optional)

Instructions:

Dough Preparation:

In a bowl, beat the egg until the white and yolk are well mixed.

Add the Oats:

Add the oats to the bowl with the beaten egg. The amount of oats can vary depending on the desired consistency. If you prefer a thicker batter, add more oats.

Season to taste:

Season the mixture with a pinch of salt (if desired) and mix well until the oats are completely incorporated into the egg.

Heat the Frying Pan:

Heat a non-stick frying pan over medium heat. There is no need to add oil as the egg and oat mixture does not stick easily.

Pour the Dough:

Pour the dough into the heated frying pan, spreading it evenly to form a little tart.

Cook over low heat:

Cook over low heat for about 2-3 minutes on each side, or until the little tart is firm and golden.

Serve with Honey and Cinnamon:

Remove the pie from the pan and place it on a plate. Drizzle with honey to taste and sprinkle with cinnamon powder.

Enjoy it:

Enjoy your egg and oat tart with honey and cinnamon as a healthy and tasty breakfast or snack.

This simple recipe is a nutritious and delicious option for a quick meal.

The honey and cinnamon add a sweet and aromatic touch to the tart, making it even tastier.

Remember to adjust the amount of oats depending on the desired dough consistency.

CARROT CAKE

Here is a simple recipe for carrot cake with sweetener and chickpea flour:

Ingredients:

FOR THE CAKE:

2 medium carrots, peeled and cut into pieces
3 eggs
1 cup sweetener of your choice (you can use culinary sweetener to taste)
1/2 cup vegetable oil (such as coconut oil or canola oil)
1 cup chickpea flour
1 teaspoon of baking powder
1 teaspoon vanilla essence (optional)
A bit of salt

FOR THE COVERAGE (OPTIONAL):

1/2 cup heavy cream (you can use light cream)
2 tablespoons powdered sweetener (or to taste)
2 tablespoons cocoa powder (optional, for a touch of
chocolate)
Chocolate or carrot shavings for decoration (optional)

Instructions:

Preparation:

Preheat the oven to 180°C. Grease and flour a cake tin
(approximately 20 cm in diameter).

Blend the Ingredients:

In a blender, place the carrots, eggs, sweetener, oil and vanilla
essence (if using). Mix until you get a smooth mixture.

Add the Dry Ingredients:

In a separate bowl, mix the chickpea flour, baking powder and
a pinch of salt. Add the dry ingredients to the liquid mixture in
the blender and blend again until all ingredients are well
combined.

Bake the Cake:

Pour the batter into the prepared pan and bake in the preheated oven for around 30-35 minutes, or until a toothpick inserted into the center comes out clean. Baking time may vary, so keep an eye on the cake.

Prepare the Cover (optional):

While the cake is baking, you can prepare the frosting. In a bowl, mix the cream, sweetener, and cocoa powder (if using). Mix well until you get a creamy coverage.

Finish the Cake:

After removing the cake from the oven and letting it cool slightly, you can spread the frosting on top, if desired. Decorate with chocolate or carrot shavings, if you prefer.

Serve and Enjoy it:

Cut the cake into slices and serve it.

This carrot cake is a healthier option, without refined sugar and with chickpea flour, making it suitable for people looking to reduce their consumption of refined carbohydrates.

Keep in mind that when using sweeteners, the sweetness can vary depending on the brand and type of sweetener you choose. Therefore, adjust the amount of sweetener according to your personal preferences.

MAIZENA PORRIDGE

You can prepare a delicious cornstarch porridge with chocolate powder to eat cold.

Here is the recipe:

Ingredients:

2 cups of milk
3 tablespoons cornstarch
2 tablespoons chocolate powder (or unsweetened cocoa powder)
1 teaspoon vanilla essence (optional)
Chocolate sprinkles (optional, for decoration)

Instructions:

Mix the Dry Ingredients:

In a bowl, mix the cornstarch, chocolate powder and sweetener. Mix well to ensure the dry ingredients are well combined.

Dissolve the cornstarch:

In a pan, pour the milk and place over medium heat. Before the milk starts to boil, slowly add the cornstarch and chocolate mixture, stirring constantly to prevent lumps from forming.

Cook until thickened:

Continue cooking the porridge over medium-low heat, stirring constantly, until it starts to thicken. This may take 5 to 10 minutes, depending on the intensity of the fire. Make sure to stir well to prevent the porridge from sticking to the bottom of the pan.

Add Vanilla Essence (optional):

If you are using vanilla essence, add it to the porridge and mix well.

Cool and Serve:

Once the porridge reaches the desired consistency (it should be very thick), remove it from the heat and let it cool slightly. Then, place it in individual pots or a larger container.

Very Cold:

To turn your porridge into a cold dessert, place it in the fridge for a few hours or until it's very cold.

Decorate and Serve:

Before serving, you can decorate with chocolate sprinkles if desired.

This cornstarch porridge with chocolate powder is a delicious and satisfying dessert that can replace higher-calorie sweets. It's creamy, has a pleasant chocolate flavor and is perfect to be consumed cold.

Enjoy it!

Here's a list of sugar-free desserts that can help satisfy your sweet tooth while you're on a healthier diet. These desserts are sweetened naturally or with sugar substitutes, making them more diet-friendly options:

Fresh fruit:

Fruits like strawberries, blueberries, raspberries, apples, pears and kiwis can be delicious desserts in their own right. Enrich with fat-free and sugar-free whipped cream.

Natural Yogurt with Fruit:

Combine plain (unsweetened) yogurt with fresh or frozen fruit for a refreshing dessert.

Fruit and Vegetable Smoothies:

Blend fruits and vegetables with water, unsweetened milk or yogurt to create healthy, sweet smoothies.

Avocado mousse:

Blend ripe avocado, unsweetened cocoa powder, almond milk, and a natural sweetener like honey or stevia to create a healthy chocolate mousse.

Chia pudding:

Mix chia seeds with unsweetened almond milk and a natural sweetener. Let it rest in the fridge until it thickens. Add fruit or vanilla extract for more flavor.

Oat and Fruit Bars:

Combine oats, unsweetened dried fruit, nuts and seeds with a little honey or maple syrup. Shape into bars and place in the fridge to harden.

Banana`s Ice-cream:

Freeze ripe bananas and then blend in a blender until you get an ice cream consistency. Add unsweetened cocoa powder or vanilla extract for extra flavor.

Açaí Bowl:

Mix frozen açaí pulp with fruit, seeds and a little honey or agave syrup. Serve as a bowl with healthy toppings.

Fruit Popsicle:

Make homemade popsicles using natural fruit juice or a sugar-free fruit smoothie.

Oatmeal and Banana Cookies:

Mix oats, mashed ripe bananas, chopped nuts and cinnamon. Bake in cookie form until golden.

Fruit Salad with Mint:

Combine a variety of fresh fruits and season with a little lemon juice and fresh mint leaves.

Fruit Compote:

Cook fresh fruit, such as apples or pears, with a little water and cinnamon until they are soft. No need to add sugar.

Yogurt Popsicle:

Mix unsweetened natural yogurt with fruit and pour into popsicle molds. Freeze until hardened.

Tofu Pudding:

Blend silken tofu with unsweetened cocoa powder, vanilla extract, and a natural sweetener. Blend until smooth and serve.

Remembering that the moderate use of natural sweeteners, such as honey, maple syrup, stevia or coconut sugar, can be an option to sweeten these sugar-free desserts. The amount of sweetener should be adjusted according to your personal preferences.

WHAT YOU SHOULD DO FROM THE MOMENT YOU START THE PATH TOWARDS YOUR GOAL OF A HEALTHY BODY:

Always think before eating.

If you're in the mood for something sweet, make something that replaces it, but made with sweetener.

Go to the supermarket with time to analyze each item and buy carefully.

We currently have 0 fat, 0 sugar options, with 100 percent flavor.

The people in your family will not need to follow the same diet as you, but they shouldn't eat sweets or all the treats that you gave up.

Rest assured about this; everyone's health will be taken care of.

Day 1:

Breakfast: Oatmeal Pie

Morning Snack: Fruits (e.g. apple)

Lunch: Quinoa with beans, sautéed vegetables (broccoli, carrots, peppers) and tuna

Dessert: yogurt with honey

Afternoon Snack: Fruits (e.g. banana)

Dinner: Quinoa with beans, green leaf salad and grilled dogfish

Dessert: fruit with honey

Meal before bed: Oat porridge or cornstarch

Note: If you are hungry during the day, you can eat fruit or yogurt with honey.

Day 2:

Breakfast: Oatmeal Pie

Morning Snack: Fruits (e.g. pear)

Lunch: Quinoa with chickpeas and sautéed vegetables (broccoli, carrots, peppers)

Afternoon Snack: Fruits (e.g. grapes)

Dinner: Quinoa with green leaf salad and grilled dogfish

Meal before bed: Oatmeal or cornstarch porridge

Note: If you are hungry during the day, you can eat fruit or yogurt with honey.

Day 3:

Breakfast: Oatmeal Pie

Morning Snack: Fruits (e.g. orange)

Lunch: Quinoa with lentils and sautéed vegetables (broccoli, carrots, peppers)

Afternoon Snack: Fruits (e.g. kiwi)

Dinner: Quinoa with vegetables and roasted dogfish

Meal before bed: Oatmeal porridge

Day 4:

Breakfast: Oatmeal Pie

Morning Snack: Fruits (e.g. banana)

Lunch: Quinoa with chickpeas and sautéed vegetables (broccoli, carrots, peppers)

Afternoon Snack: Fruits (e.g. apple)

Dinner: Quinoa with green leaf salad and grilled dogfish

Meal before bed: Cornstarch Porridge

Day 5:

Breakfast: Oatmeal Pie

Morning Snack: Fruits (e.g. pear)

Lunch: Quinoa with lentils and sautéed vegetables (broccoli, carrots, peppers)

Afternoon Snack: Fruits (e.g. grapes)

Dinner: Quinoa with vegetables and roasted dogfish

Meal before bed: Oatmeal Porridge

Day 6:

Breakfast: Oatmeal Pie

Morning Snack: Fruits (e.g. orange)

Lunch: Quinoa with chickpeas and sautéed vegetables (broccoli, carrots, peppers)

Afternoon Snack: Fruits (e.g. kiwi)

Dinner: Quinoa with green leaf salad and grilled dogfish

Meal before bed: Oatmeal Porridge

Day 7:

Breakfast: Oatmeal Pie

Morning Snack: Fruits (e.g. banana)

Lunch: Quinoa with lentils and sautéed vegetables (broccoli, carrots, peppers)

Afternoon Snack: Fruits (e.g. apple)

Dinner: Quinoa with vegetables and roasted dogfish

Meal before bed: Cornstarch Porridge

Day 8:

Breakfast: Oatmeal Pie

Morning Snack: Fruits (e.g. pear)

Lunch: Quinoa with chickpeas and sautéed vegetables (broccoli, carrots, peppers)

Afternoon Snack: Fruits (e.g. grapes)

Dinner: Quinoa with green leaf salad and grilled dogfish

Meal before bed: Oatmeal Porridge

Day 9:

Breakfast: Oatmeal Pie

Morning Snack: Fruits (e.g. orange)

Lunch: Quinoa with lentils and sautéed vegetables (broccoli, carrots, peppers)

Afternoon Snack: Fruits (e.g. kiwi)

Dinner: Quinoa with vegetables and roasted dogfish

Meal before bed: Oatmeal Porridge

Day 10:

Breakfast: Oatmeal Pie

Morning Snack: Fruits (e.g. banana)

Lunch: Quinoa with chickpeas and sautéed vegetables (broccoli, carrots, peppers)

Afternoon Snack: Fruits (e.g. apple)

Dinner: Quinoa with green leaf salad and grilled dogfish

Meal before bed: Cornstarch Porridge

Day 11:

Breakfast: Oatmeal Pie

Morning Snack: Fruits (e.g. pear)

Lunch: Quinoa with lentils and sautéed vegetables (broccoli, carrots, peppers)

Afternoon Snack: Fruits (e.g. grapes)

Dinner: Quinoa with green leaf salad and grilled dogfish

Meal before bed: Oatmeal Porridge

Evening Tea: Chamomile

If you're hungry: Carrots

Day 12:

Breakfast: Oatmeal Pie

Morning Snack: Fruits (e.g. orange)

Lunch: Quinoa with chickpeas and sautéed vegetables (broccoli, carrots, peppers)

Afternoon Snack: Fruits (e.g. kiwi)

Dinner: Quinoa with vegetables and roasted dogfish

Meal before bed: Oatmeal Porridge

Evening Tea: Mint

If you're hungry: Carrots

Day 13:

Breakfast: Oatmeal Pie

Morning Snack: Fruits (e.g. banana)

Lunch: Quinoa with lentils and sautéed vegetables (broccoli, carrots, peppers)

Afternoon Snack: Fruits (e.g. apple)

Dinner: Quinoa with green leaf salad and grilled dogfish

Meal before bed: Cornstarch Porridge

Evening Tea: Lemon Balm

If you're hungry: Carrots

Day 14:

Breakfast: Oatmeal Pie

Morning Snack: Fruits (e.g. pear)

Lunch: Quinoa with chickpeas and sautéed vegetables (broccoli, carrots, peppers)

Afternoon Snack: Fruits (e.g. grapes)

Dinner: Quinoa with vegetables and roasted dogfish

Meal before bed: Oatmeal Porridge

Evening Tea: Green Tea

If you're hungry: Carrots

Day 15:

Breakfast: Oatmeal Pie

Morning Snack: Fruits (e.g. orange)

Lunch: Quinoa with lentils and sautéed vegetables (broccoli, carrots, peppers)

Afternoon Snack: Fruits (e.g. kiwi)

Dinner: Quinoa with green leaf salad and grilled dogfish

Meal before bed: Oatmeal Porridge

Evening Tea: Ginger

If you're hungry: Carrots

Day 16:

Breakfast: Oatmeal Pie

Morning Snack: Fruits (e.g. banana)

Lunch: Quinoa with chickpeas and sautéed vegetables (broccoli, carrots, peppers)

Afternoon Snack: Fruits (e.g. apple)

Dinner: Quinoa with vegetables and roasted dogfish

Meal before bed: Cornstarch Porridge

Evening Tea: Cinnamon Tea

If you're hungry: Carrots

Day 17:

Breakfast: Oatmeal Pie

Morning Snack: Fruits (e.g. pear)

Lunch: Quinoa with lentils and sautéed vegetables (broccoli, carrots, peppers)

Afternoon Snack: Fruits (e.g. grapes)

Dinner: Quinoa with green leaf salad and grilled dogfish

Meal before bed: Oatmeal Porridge

Evening Tea: Apple Tea

If you're hungry: Carrots

Day 18:

Breakfast: Oatmeal Pie

Morning Snack: Fruits (e.g. orange)

Lunch: Quinoa with chickpeas and sautéed vegetables (broccoli, carrots, peppers)

Afternoon Snack: Fruits (e.g. kiwi)

Dinner: Quinoa with vegetables and roasted dogfish

Meal before bed: Oatmeal Porridge

Evening Tea: Chamomile Tea

If you're hungry: Carrots

Day 19:

Breakfast: Oatmeal Pie

Morning Snack: Fruits (e.g. banana)

Lunch: Quinoa with lentils and sautéed vegetables (broccoli, carrots, peppers)

Afternoon Snack: Fruits (e.g. apple)

Dinner: Quinoa with green leaf salad and grilled dogfish

Meal before bed: Cornstarch Porridge

Evening Tea: Lavender Tea

If you're hungry: Carrots

Day 20:

Breakfast: Oatmeal Pie

Morning Snack: Fruits (e.g. pear)

Lunch: Quinoa with chickpeas and sautéed vegetables (broccoli, carrots, peppers)

Afternoon Snack: Fruits (e.g. grapes)

Dinner: Quinoa with vegetables and roasted dogfish

Meal before bed: Oatmeal Porridge

Evening Tea: Lemon Balm Tea

If you're hungry: Carrots

Day 21:

Breakfast: Oatmeal Pie

Morning Snack: Fruits (e.g. orange)

Lunch: Quinoa with lentils and sautéed vegetables (broccoli, carrots, peppers)

Afternoon Snack: Fruits (e.g. kiwi)

Dinner: Quinoa with vegetables and roasted dogfish

Meal before bed: Oatmeal Porridge

Evening Tea: Ginger Tea

If you're hungry: Carrots

Day 22:

Breakfast: Oatmeal Pie

Morning Snack: Fruits (e.g. banana)

Lunch: Quinoa with chickpeas and sautéed vegetables (broccoli, carrots, peppers)

Afternoon Snack: Fruits (e.g. apple)

Dinner: Quinoa with green leaf salad and grilled dogfish

Meal before bed: Cornstarch Porridge

Evening Tea: Chamomile Tea

If you're hungry: Carrots

Day 23:

Breakfast: Oatmeal Pie

Morning Snack: Fruits (e.g. pear)

Lunch: Quinoa with lentils and sautéed vegetables (broccoli, carrots, peppers)

Afternoon Snack: Fruits (e.g. grapes)

Dinner: Quinoa with vegetables and roasted dogfish

Meal before bed: Oatmeal Porridge

Evening Tea: Lavender Tea

If you're hungry: Carrots

Day 24:

Breakfast: Oatmeal Pie

Morning Snack: Fruits (e.g. orange)

Lunch: Quinoa with chickpeas and sautéed vegetables (broccoli, carrots, peppers)

Afternoon Snack: Fruits (e.g. kiwi)

Dinner: Quinoa with green leaf salad and grilled dogfish

Meal before bed: Oatmeal Porridge

Evening Tea: Green Tea

If you're hungry: Carrots

Day 25:

Breakfast: Oatmeal Pie

Morning Snack: Fruits (e.g. banana)

Lunch: Quinoa with lentils and sautéed vegetables (broccoli, carrots, peppers)

Afternoon Snack: Fruits (e.g. apple)

Dinner: Quinoa with vegetables and roasted dogfish

Meal before bed: Cornstarch Porridge

Evening Tea: Lemon Balm Tea

If you're hungry: Carrots

Day 26:

Breakfast: Oatmeal Pie

Morning Snack: Fruits (e.g. pear)

Lunch: Quinoa with chickpeas and sautéed vegetables (broccoli, carrots, peppers)

Afternoon Snack: Fruits (e.g. grapes)

Dinner: Quinoa with green leaf salad and grilled dogfish

Meal before bed: Oatmeal Porridge

Evening Tea: Apple Tea

If you're hungry: Carrots

Day 27:

Breakfast: Oatmeal Pie

Morning Snack: Fruits (e.g. orange)

Lunch: Quinoa with lentils and sautéed vegetables (broccoli, carrots, peppers)

Afternoon Snack: Fruits (e.g. kiwi)

Dinner: Quinoa with vegetables and roasted dogfish

Meal before bed: Oatmeal Porridge

Evening Tea: Cinnamon Tea

If you're hungry: Carrots

<h1 style="text-align:center">Day 28:</h1>

Breakfast: Oatmeal Pie

Morning Snack: Fruits (e.g. banana)

Lunch: Quinoa with chickpeas and sautéed vegetables (broccoli, carrots, peppers)

Afternoon Snack: Fruits (e.g. apple)

Dinner: Quinoa with green leaf salad and grilled dogfish

Meal before bed: Cornstarch Porridge

Evening Tea: Lavender Tea

If you're hungry: Carrots

Day 29:

Breakfast: Oatmeal Pie

Morning Snack: Fruits (e.g. pear)

Lunch: Quinoa with lentils and sautéed vegetables (broccoli, carrots, peppers)

Afternoon Snack: Fruits (e.g. grapes)

Dinner: Quinoa with vegetables and roasted dogfish

Meal before bed: Oatmeal Porridge

Evening Tea: Ginger Tea

If you're hungry: Carrots

Day 30:

Breakfast: Oatmeal Pie

Morning Snack: Fruits (e.g. orange)

Lunch: Quinoa with chickpeas and sautéed vegetables (broccoli, carrots, peppers)

Afternoon Snack: Fruits (e.g. kiwi)

Dinner: Quinoa with green leaf salad and grilled dogfish

Meal before bed: Oatmeal Porridge

Evening Tea: Chamomile Tea

If you're hungry: Carrots

Day 31:

Breakfast: Oatmeal Pie

Morning Snack: Fruits (e.g. banana)

Lunch: Quinoa with lentils and sautéed vegetables (broccoli, carrots, peppers)

Afternoon Snack: Fruits (e.g. apple)

Dinner: Quinoa with vegetables and roasted dogfish

Meal before bed: Cornstarch Porridge

Evening Tea: Lemon Balm Tea

If you're hungry: Carrots

YOU MADE IT THIS FAR!!!

TODAY IS THE DAY TO MEASURE YOUR VICTORIES.

Date____/____/____

Neck:

Bust:

Waist:

Hip:

Right arm:

Left arm:

Right thigh:

Left thigh:

Do this every month and be happy with the results.

FROM NOW ON, FOR GREATER VITAMIN CARE

YOU'RE READY TO ADD THE JUICE DIET TO THIS PROGRAM.

BOOK AT YOUR DISPOSAL, AT

AMAZON.COM

"THE MAGIC JUICE"
AUTHOR: A.L.R.B.

Series: Healthy Eating

Day 32:

Breakfast: Oatmeal Pie

Morning Snack: Fruits (e.g. orange)

Lunch: Quinoa with lentils and sautéed vegetables (broccoli, carrots, peppers)

Afternoon Snack: Fruits (e.g. kiwi)

Dinner: Quinoa with vegetables and roasted dogfish

Meal before bed: Oatmeal Porridge

Evening Tea: Ginger Tea

If you're hungry: Carrots

Day 33:

Breakfast: Oatmeal Pie

Morning Snack: Fruits (e.g. banana)

Lunch: Quinoa with chickpeas and sautéed vegetables (broccoli, carrots, peppers)

Afternoon Snack: Fruits (e.g. apple)

Dinner: Quinoa with green leaf salad and grilled dogfish

Meal before bed: Cornstarch Porridge

Evening Tea: Chamomile Tea

If you're hungry: Carrots

Day 34:

Breakfast: Oatmeal Pie

Morning Snack: Fruits (e.g. pear)

Lunch: Quinoa with lentils and sautéed vegetables (broccoli, carrots, peppers)

Afternoon Snack: Fruits (e.g. grapes)

Dinner: Quinoa with vegetables and roasted dogfish

Meal before bed: Oatmeal Porridge

Evening Tea: Lavender Tea

If you're hungry: Carrots

Day 35:

Breakfast: Oatmeal Pie

Morning Snack: Fruits (e.g. orange)

Lunch: Quinoa with chickpeas and sautéed vegetables (broccoli, carrots, peppers)

Afternoon Snack: Fruits (e.g. kiwi)

Dinner: Quinoa with green leaf salad and grilled dogfish

Meal before bed: Oatmeal Porridge

Evening Tea: Green Tea

If you're hungry: Carrots

Day 36:

Breakfast: Oatmeal Pie

Morning Snack: Fruits (e.g. banana)

Lunch: Quinoa with lentils and sautéed vegetables (broccoli, carrots, peppers)

Afternoon Snack: Fruits (e.g. apple)

Dinner: Quinoa with vegetables and roasted dogfish

Meal before bed: Cornstarch Porridge

Evening Tea: Lemon Balm Tea

If you're hungry: Carrots

Day 37:

Breakfast: Oatmeal Pie

Morning Snack: Fruits (e.g. pear)

Lunch: Quinoa with chickpeas and sautéed vegetables (broccoli, carrots, peppers)

Afternoon Snack: Fruits (e.g. grapes)

Dinner: Quinoa with vegetables and roasted dogfish

Meal before bed: Oatmeal Porridge

Evening Tea: Apple Tea

If you're hungry: Carrots

Day 38:

Breakfast: Oatmeal Pie

Morning Snack: Fruits (e.g. orange)

Lunch: Quinoa with lentils and sautéed vegetables (broccoli, carrots, peppers)

Afternoon Snack: Fruits (e.g. kiwi)

Dinner: Quinoa with green leaf salad and grilled dogfish

Meal before bed: Oatmeal Porridge

Evening Tea: Cinnamon Tea

If you're hungry: Carrots

Day 39:

Breakfast: Oatmeal Pie

Morning Snack: Fruits (e.g. banana)

Lunch: Quinoa with chickpeas and sautéed vegetables (broccoli, carrots, peppers)

Afternoon Snack: Fruits (e.g. apple)

Dinner: Quinoa with vegetables and roasted dogfish

Meal before bed: Cornstarch Porridge

Evening Tea: Lavender Tea

If you're hungry: Carrots

Day 40:

Breakfast: Oatmeal Pie

Morning Snack: Fruits (e.g. pear)

Lunch: Quinoa with lentils and sautéed vegetables (broccoli, carrots, peppers)

Afternoon Snack: Fruits (e.g. grapes)

Dinner: Quinoa with vegetables and roasted dogfish

Meal before bed: Oatmeal Porridge

Evening Tea: Ginger Tea

If you're hungry: Carrots

Day 41:

Breakfast: Oatmeal Pie

Morning Snack: Fruits (e.g. orange)

Lunch: Quinoa with chickpeas and sautéed vegetables (broccoli, carrots, peppers)

Afternoon Snack: Fruits (e.g. kiwi)

Dinner: Quinoa with green leaf salad and grilled dogfish

Meal before bed: Oatmeal Porridge

Evening Tea: Chamomile Tea

If you're hungry: Carrots

Day 42:

Breakfast: Oatmeal Pie

Morning Snack: Fruits (e.g. banana)

Lunch: Quinoa with lentils and sautéed vegetables (broccoli, carrots, peppers)

Afternoon Snack: Fruits (e.g. apple)

Dinner: Quinoa with vegetables and roasted dogfish

Meal before bed: Cornstarch Porridge

Evening Tea: Lemon Balm Tea

If you're hungry: Carrots

Day 43:

Breakfast: Oatmeal pie and 2 boiled eggs

Morning Snack: Fruits (e.g. orange)

Lunch: Quinoa with lentils, sautéed vegetables (broccoli, carrots, peppers) and grilled chicken breast

Afternoon Snack: Fruits (e.g. kiwi)

Dinner: Quinoa with vegetables and roasted dogfish

Meal before bed: Cornstarch Porridge

Evening Tea: Chamomile Tea

If you're hungry: Carrots

Day 44:

Breakfast: Oatmeal pie and spinach omelet with 2 eggs

Morning Snack: Fruits (e.g. banana)

Lunch: Quinoa with lentils, sautéed vegetables (broccoli, carrots, peppers) and grilled chicken breast

Afternoon Snack: Fruits (e.g. apple)

Dinner: Quinoa with vegetables and chicken fillet in lemon sauce

Meal before bed: Oatmeal Porridge

Evening Tea: Green Tea

If you're hungry: Carrots

Day 45:

Breakfast: Oatmeal pie and scrambled eggs with spinach

Morning Snack: Fruits (e.g. pear)

Lunch: Quinoa with lentils, sautéed vegetables (broccoli, carrots, peppers) and grilled chicken breast

Afternoon Snack: Fruits (e.g. grapes)

Dinner: Quinoa with vegetables and grilled chicken fillet

Meal before bed: Oatmeal Porridge

Evening Tea: Lavender Tea

If you're hungry: Carrots

Day 46:

Breakfast: Oatmeal pie and 2 boiled eggs

Morning Snack: Fruits (e.g. orange)

Lunch: Quinoa with lentils, sautéed vegetables (broccoli, carrots, peppers) and grilled chicken breast

Afternoon Snack: Fruits (e.g. kiwi)

Dinner: Quinoa with vegetables and chicken fillet in mustard sauce

Meal before bed: Cornstarch Porridge

Evening Tea: Chamomile Tea

If you're hungry: Carrots

Day 47:

Breakfast: Oatmeal pie and spinach omelet with 2 eggs

Morning Snack: Fruits (e.g. banana)

Lunch: Quinoa with lentils, sautéed vegetables (broccoli, carrots, peppers) and grilled chicken breast

Afternoon Snack: Fruits (e.g. apple)

Dinner: Quinoa with vegetables and grilled chicken breast

Meal before bed: Oatmeal Porridge

Evening Tea: Green Tea

If you're hungry: Carrots

Day 48:

Breakfast: Oatmeal pie and scrambled eggs with spinach

Morning Snack: Fruits (e.g. pear)

Lunch: Quinoa with lentils, sautéed vegetables (broccoli, carrots, peppers) and grilled chicken breast

Afternoon Snack: Fruits (e.g. grapes)

Dinner: Quinoa with vegetables and chicken fillet in lemon sauce

Meal before bed: Cornstarch Porridge

Evening Tea: Lavender Tea

If you're hungry: Carrots

Day 49:

Breakfast: Oatmeal pie and 2 boiled eggs

Morning Snack: Fruits (e.g. orange)

Lunch: Quinoa with lentils, sautéed vegetables (broccoli, carrots, peppers) and grilled chicken breast

Afternoon Snack: Fruits (e.g. kiwi)

Dinner: Quinoa with vegetables and chicken fillet in mustard sauce

Meal before bed: Oatmeal Porridge

Evening Tea: Chamomile Tea

If you're hungry: Carrots

Day 50:

Breakfast: Oatmeal pie and spinach omelet with 2 eggs

Morning Snack: Fruits (e.g. banana)

Lunch: Quinoa with lentils, sautéed vegetables (broccoli, carrots, peppers) and grilled chicken breast

Afternoon Snack: Fruits (e.g. apple)

Dinner: Quinoa with vegetables and grilled chicken breast

Meal before bed: Cornstarch Porridge

Evening Tea: Green Tea

If you're hungry: Carrots

Day 51:

Breakfast: Oatmeal pie and scrambled eggs with spinach

Morning Snack: Fruits (e.g. pear)

Lunch: Quinoa with lentils, sautéed vegetables (broccoli, carrots, peppers) and grilled chicken breast

Afternoon Snack: Fruits (e.g. grapes)

Dinner: Quinoa with vegetables and chicken fillet in lemon sauce

Meal before bed: Cornstarch Porridge

Evening Tea: Lavender Tea

If you're hungry: Carrots

Day 52:

Breakfast: Oatmeal pie and 2 boiled eggs

Morning Snack: Fruits (e.g. orange)

Lunch: Quinoa with lentils, sautéed vegetables (broccoli, carrots, peppers) and grilled chicken breast

Afternoon Snack: Fruits (e.g. kiwi)

Dinner: Quinoa with vegetables and chicken fillet in mustard sauce

Meal before bed: Oatmeal Porridge

Evening Tea: Chamomile Tea

If you're hungry: Carrots

Day 53:

Breakfast: Oatmeal pie and spinach omelet with 2 eggs

Morning Snack: Fruits (e.g. banana)

Lunch: Quinoa with lentils, sautéed vegetables (broccoli, carrots, peppers) and grilled chicken breast

Afternoon Snack: Fruits (e.g. apple)

Dinner: Quinoa with vegetables and grilled chicken breast

Meal before bed: Cornstarch Porridge

Evening Tea: Green Tea

If you're hungry: Carrots

Day 54:

Breakfast: Oatmeal pie and scrambled eggs with spinach

Morning Snack: Fruits (e.g. pear)

Lunch: Quinoa with lentils, sautéed vegetables (broccoli, carrots, peppers) and grilled chicken breast

Afternoon Snack: Fruits (e.g. grapes)

Dinner: Quinoa with vegetables and chicken fillet in lemon sauce

Meal before bed: Cornstarch Porridge

Evening Tea: Lavender Tea

If you're hungry: Carrots

Day 55:

Breakfast: Oatmeal pie and 2 boiled eggs

Morning Snack: Fruits (e.g. orange)

Lunch: Quinoa with lentils, sautéed vegetables (broccoli, carrots, peppers) and grilled chicken breast

Afternoon Snack: Fruits (e.g. kiwi)

Dinner: Quinoa with vegetables and chicken fillet in mustard sauce

Meal before bed: Oatmeal Porridge

Evening Tea: Chamomile Tea

If you're hungry: Carrots

Day 56:

Breakfast: Oatmeal pie and spinach omelet with 2 eggs

Morning Snack: Fruits (e.g. banana)

Lunch: Quinoa with lentils, sautéed vegetables (broccoli, carrots, peppers) and grilled chicken breast

Afternoon Snack: Fruits (e.g. apple)

Dinner: Quinoa with vegetables and grilled chicken fillet

Meal before bed: Cornstarch Porridge

Evening Tea: Green Tea

If you're hungry: Carrots

Day 57:

Breakfast: Oatmeal pie and scrambled eggs with spinach

Morning Snack: Fruits (e.g. pear)

Lunch: Quinoa with lentils, sautéed vegetables (broccoli, carrots, peppers) and grilled chicken breast

Afternoon Snack: Fruits (e.g. grapes)

Dinner: Quinoa with vegetables and chicken fillet in lemon sauce

Meal before bed: Cornstarch Porridge

Evening Tea: Lavender Tea

If you're hungry: Carrots

Day 58:

Breakfast: Oatmeal pie and 2 boiled eggs

Morning Snack: Fruits (e.g. orange)

Lunch: Quinoa with lentils, sautéed vegetables (broccoli, carrots, peppers) and grilled chicken breast

Afternoon Snack: Fruits (e.g. kiwi)

Dinner: Quinoa with vegetables and chicken fillet in mustard sauce

Meal before bed: Oatmeal Porridge

Evening Tea: Chamomile Tea

If you're hungry: Carrots

Day 59:

Breakfast: Oatmeal pie and spinach omelet with 2 eggs

Morning Snack: Fruits (e.g. banana)

Lunch: Quinoa with lentils, sautéed vegetables (broccoli, carrots, peppers) and grilled chicken breast

Afternoon Snack: Fruits (e.g. apple)

Dinner: Quinoa with vegetables and grilled chicken fillet

Meal before bed: Cornstarch Porridge

Evening Tea: Green Tea

If you're hungry: Carrots

Day 60:

Breakfast: Oatmeal pie and scrambled eggs with spinach

Morning Snack: Fruits (e.g. pear)

Lunch: Quinoa with lentils, sautéed vegetables (broccoli, carrots, peppers) and grilled chicken breast

Afternoon Snack: Fruits (e.g. grapes)

Dinner: Quinoa with vegetables and chicken fillet in lemon sauce

Meal before bed: Cornstarch Porridge

Evening Tea: Lavender Tea

If you're hungry: Carrots

FROM NOW ON,

ADD SEVERAL TEAS TO YOUR LIFE.

BOOK AT YOUR DISPOSAL, AT

AMAZON.COM

"THE MAGIC TEA"

AUTHOR: A.L.R.B.

Series: Healthy Eating

THE DAY OF TODAY WILL BE DEDICATED TO FRUITS.

Day 61:

Breakfast: Various fruits (e.g. banana, apple, kiwi)

Morning Snack: Various fruits (e.g. orange, grapes)

Lunch: Fruit salad with yogurt

Afternoon Snack: Various fruits (e.g. strawberries, pineapple)

Dinner: Various fruits (e.g. watermelon, mango)

Meal before bed: Various fruits (e.g. pear, plum)

Evening Tea: Tea with your favorite fruit

If you are hungry: Various fruits (e.g. apple, banana)

FROM NOW ON

REPEAT FROM DAY 1, ADDING JUICES AND TEAS

The presented menus are suggestions to guide your diet.

You have the flexibility to choose foods you prefer, as long as they are consumed in moderation and are within the list of permitted foods.

Remember to focus on food variety and quality, prioritizing fruits, vegetables, lean proteins and whole grains.

Respect your body and your individual needs, adapting the plan according to your routine and preferences.

The key is to make conscious choices to maintain a balanced and healthy lifestyle.

"LIST OF STRICTLY PROHIBIT"

Sweets and Treats:
Cakes, cookies, ice cream, chocolates, etc.

Sugary Drinks:
Soft drinks, processed fruit juices, energy drinks, etc.

Fried and Fatty Foods:
French fries, snacks, breaded foods, etc.

Processed Meats:
Sausage, ham, bacon etc.

Fast Food:
Burgers, pizzas, hamburgers, fries etc.

Foods Rich in Saturated Fats:
Butter, fatty cheeses, red meat with visible fat, pork, etc.

Foods with High Salt Content:
Industrialized snacks, concentrated broths, canned foods, etc.

Alcoholic beverages:
Excessive alcohol can have negative impacts on
health.

Soft drinks and sweet drinks:
High in added sugars and empty calories.

Ultra-processed foods:
Industrialized products with many chemical additives
and low nutritional value.

White rice:
White rice has low nutritional value and a high
glycemic index.

Breads and Cookies:
White breads and crackers, including savory ones,
have low nutritional value and a high content of
sugars and/or harmful fats.

Toast:
Toast, being a form of bread, is also included in the
list of foods to avoid.

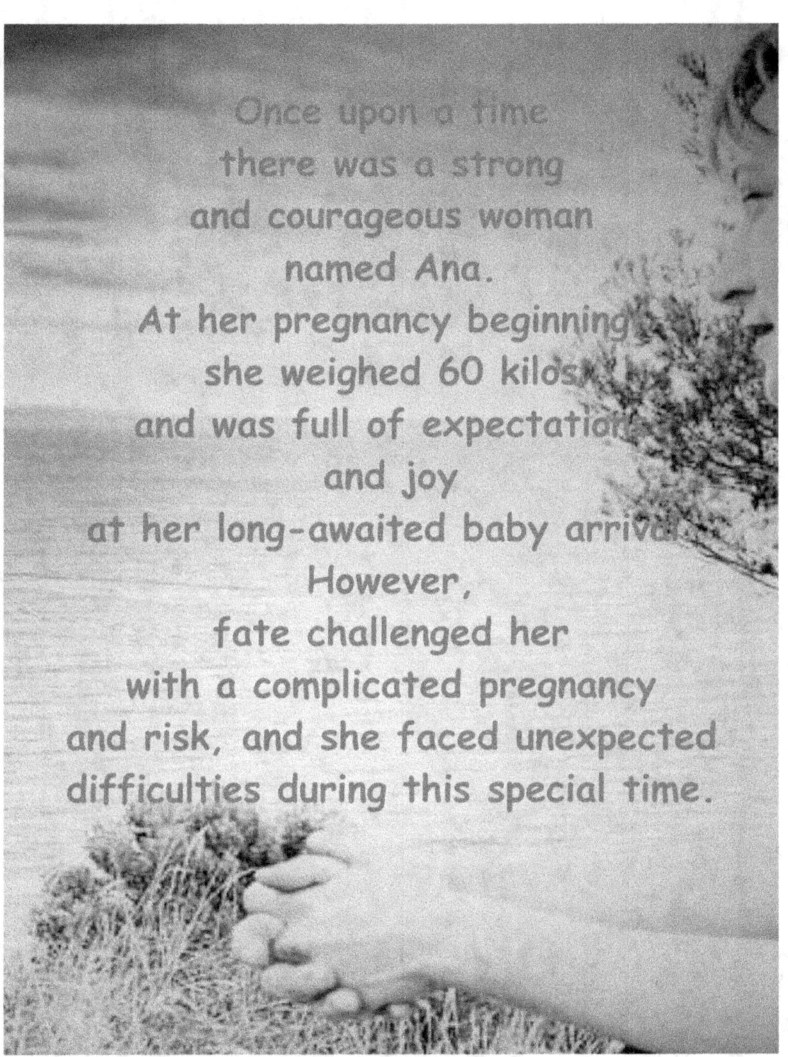

Once upon a time
there was a strong
and courageous woman
named Ana.
At her pregnancy beginning
she weighed 60 kilos
and was full of expectation
and joy
at her long-awaited baby arrival.
However,
fate challenged her
with a complicated pregnancy
and risk, and she faced unexpected
difficulties during this special time.

the months passed,
Ana's health became more fragile,
and the extra pounds
started to accumulate.
On the day of her baby birth
Ana weighed 125 kilos,
and the smile that once
adorned her face
had given way to deep sadness.
She found herself the subject of
laughter and judgmental looks,
even from her own husband,
which increased even more
her pain.

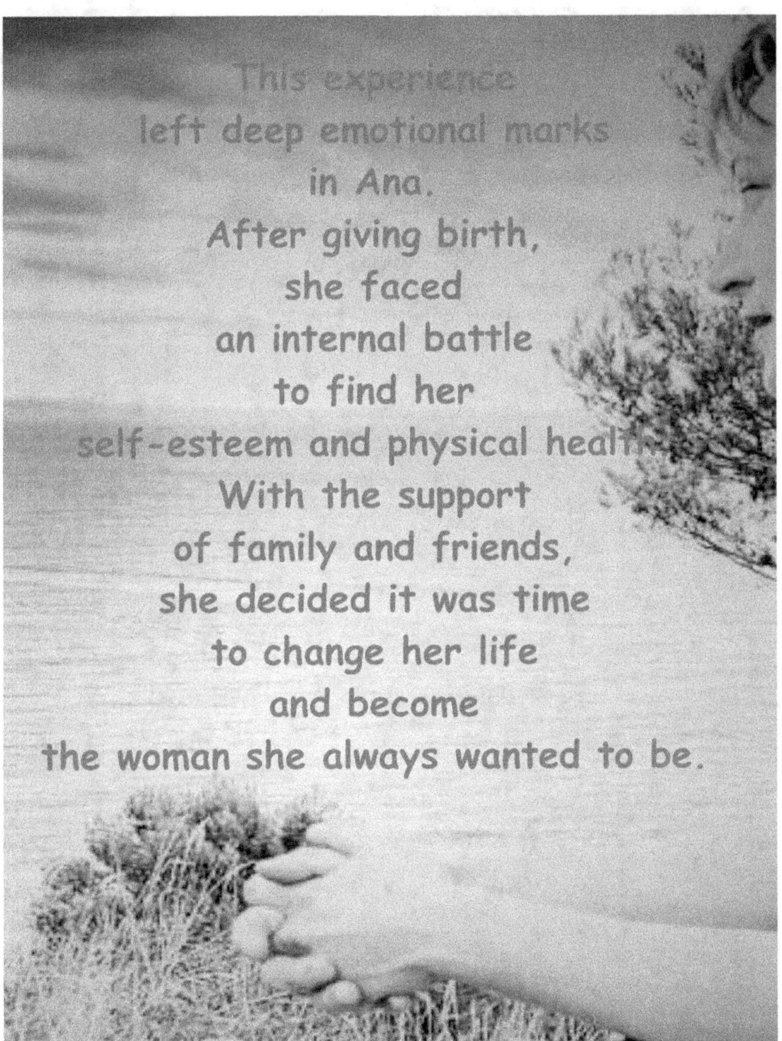
This experience
left deep emotional marks
in Ana.
After giving birth,
she faced
an internal battle
to find her
self-esteem and physical health.
With the support
of family and friends,
she decided it was time
to change her life
and become
the woman she always wanted to be.

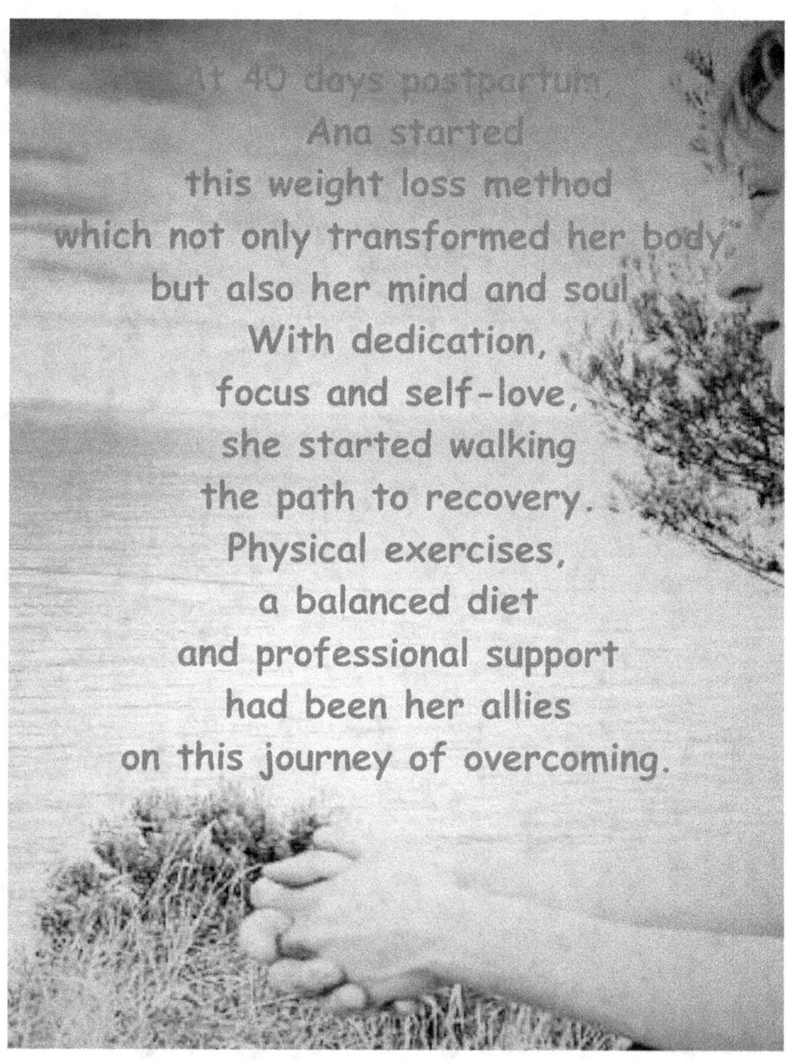

At 40 days postpartum,
Ana started
this weight loss method
which not only transformed her body,
but also her mind and soul.
With dedication,
focus and self-love,
she started walking
the path to recovery.
Physical exercises,
a balanced diet
and professional support
had been her allies
on this journey of overcoming.

er the course of a year,
Ana passed
for an incredible transformation.
She not only recovered
her pre-pregnancy body,
she also won
an indomitable inner strength.
Her emotional intelligence
became stronger,
and she learned to
value herself
and believe in her own potential.
Ana was full,
happy
and above all, healthy.

This journey
wasn't just
about weight loss,
but about gaining trust,
self-love and resilience.
Ana became an example
of determination and overcoming
to everyone around her.
Her inspiring story
showed that, with persistence
and self-love, it's possible
overcome challenges and achieve
complete happiness. And so,
Ana became the personification
of feminine strength and the human
capacity to rise again
in the face of adversity.

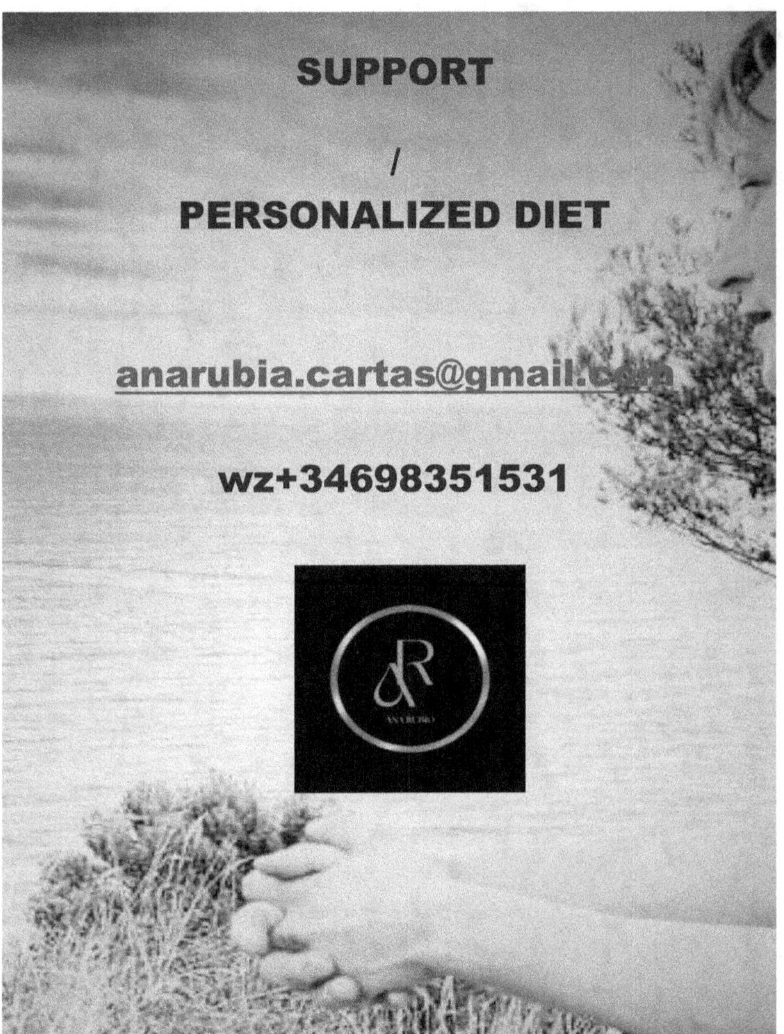
SUPPORT
/
PERSONALIZED DIET

anarubia.cartas@gmail.com

wz+34698351531